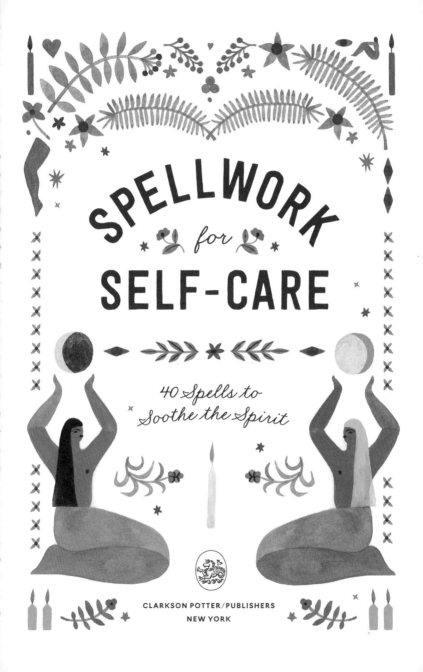

SPELLWORK *for* SELF-CARE

40 Spells to Soothe the Spirit

CLARKSON POTTER/PUBLISHERS
NEW YORK

This book is intended for informational and entertainment purposes only and is not meant to take the place of medical advice. You should consult with a medical professional before embarking on any regimen that affects your health.

Contents

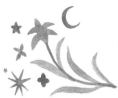

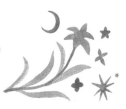

SELF-CARE

is

FEMINIST

♥

"Caring for myself is not
self-indulgence, it is
self-preservation, and that is
an act of political warfare."

—AUDRE LORDE

Self-care is about a lot more than bubble baths. Even when the action is as minor as taking half a day off for mental health, caring for yourself is a small, one-person, feminist rebellion. Many people—women especially—try to justify self-care as a way of replenishing energy so they are available to give more of themselves to other people. Having more energy to spread love and kindness is a wonderful side effect of self-care, but it is not the purpose. You do not need an excuse to take care of yourself.

Your self-care is about *you*.

For centuries, the role of women, especially women of color, has been to take care of others. Women have been raised for generations to behave as wives, mothers, and caregivers first. Not only are we expected to do all of this service and emotional labor, but we are expected to do it for free. And though women are culturally expected to read and process other people's emotions more readily than men are, our *own* pain and emotional needs are not taken seriously. The idea of women caring for themselves (and only for themselves) in an effective

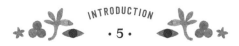

way is a very new concept. When you take the time to care for yourself, you acknowledge the inherent value of your energy, your pain, your emotions, and your body. You acknowledge that you have a *self*, a beingness outside of what you do for others. You preserve and develop that self by caring for you.

Little by little, the world can change because you value and care for yourself. As you stay mentally, emotionally, and physically healthy, you become more authentic. You learn to appreciate yourself more and demand the time, money, and love you deserve. Other people—men *and* womxn, including trans and gender-nonconforming folx—will see your hard work and feel inspired to do more for their own self-care. Person by person, the change spreads. This is how self-care stretches beyond indulgence and even self-preservation to become political and feminist—a part of the world's greater healing.

⚹ ⚹ ✦

OKAY, BUT WHY WITCHCRAFT?

Witches are wise in the ways of self-care. The craft of the wise is full of healing remedies for body, mind, and spirit. In witchcraft, there is reverence for the divine feminine and for the divine within everyone. Witches have respect for the feminine, for the divine masculine, for girls and women of all ages, and for the natural world. All of this is integral to the way you care for yourself as a divine spark in a larger web of interconnected life.

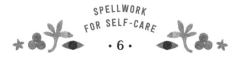

DO I HAVE TO BE WICCAN?

The community of people who practice magic is large and diverse. Even within the popular religion of Wicca, there are different traditions. Other spiritual and magical paths include, but are not limited to, Santeria, hoodoo, Druidry, eclectic paganism, ceremonial magic, chaos magic, and various forms of traditional witchcraft. Some magical practitioners have relationships to gods and/or goddesses and others do not. These spells are not designed for any particular spiritual or magical path; what they have in common is their intent for self-care.

✳ ✳ ✦

WHAT IS MAGIC?

A creative director is branding a new sneaker company. He gives the business a name, chooses a color palette, and has a logo designed, all for the specific, intended effect of attracting a young audience. He chooses a special date for the launch and invites the right influential people to support the business. Together with his team, he develops advertisements that tell a story about the incomparable speed, comfort, and coolness of the company's shoes. When the branding campaign is a success, the company sees profits immediately.

A witch is looking for love. She chooses colors and symbols for the spell that will produce the specific, intended effect of finding love. She chooses the right date for her spellwork based on the

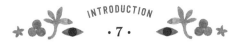

movements of the moon and invites the right influential spirits to help support her intention. She develops a story about the qualities her ideal partner will possess and what the relationship will look like. The spell is a success: the witch meets someone who has the qualities she's looking for.

Which of them used magic to get what they wanted?

Magic is the effect of your will on the world, aided by the use of the symbolic. If you're willing to suspend disbelief and work your own will on the world, magic is yours for the taking. When used properly, magic becomes a spiritual campaign for your own success and happiness. It is the work of your focused intention, but it also reaches beyond you.

There are other forces at work besides your will. Some will help you and some will harm you if you aren't careful. These forces include spirits such as angels, demons, saints, fairies, ghosts, and gods. It's important to remember that you are interacting with the unseen world and to protect yourself accordingly. Some of the spells in this book call on specific goddesses, gods, and planets, but most don't. You may adapt spells according to your spiritual tradition, including the deities and spirits you feel called into relationship with.

It's also important to remember that while magic can aid you in your endeavors, it does not do everything for you. You are still responsible for your decisions in everyday life. Casting a psychic shield or carrying a talisman, for example, does not empower you

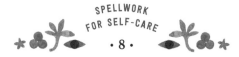

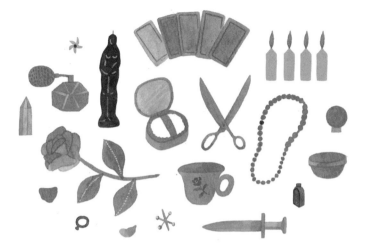

to seek out dangerous situations. Protective magic increases the power of your personal force field to help ward danger away. It does not make you invincible. Always take basic precautions for your safety regardless of the magic you're using.

The ingredients of magic are all around you. They're in your spice cabinet, your garden, your jewelry, the colors you wear, and the perfume you like. Selecting specific ingredients, and putting them together with intention, is what witches call spellwork. It brings the magic within you and the magic around you into harmony, producing remarkable results.

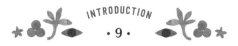

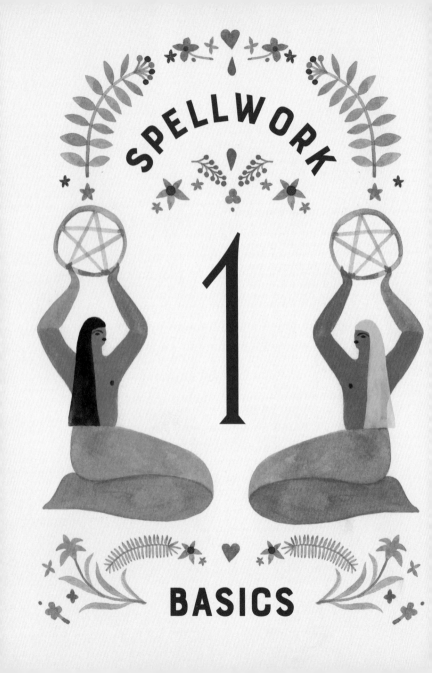

SPELLWORK

1

BASICS

Spellwork is the work involved in doing magic in a particular way for effect. It is "work" because it often requires you to gather specific materials ahead of time, set aside time for your spellwork, and then make, write, burn, or bury something. A few of the spells in this book require only your imagination, while others come with a list of ingredients to gather. The gathering is part of your spellwork. Witches and other magical practitioners often call a spell in progress a "working." If doing magic were easy, everyone would cast spells.

Some say you don't need spells to do magic. You don't need candlelight, or herbs, or crystals, or essential oils, or squiggly symbols, or Latin words. There is a truth there: at the heart of magic, technically all you need is clear, thoughtful intention. But the difference between a deliberate thought and a spell is the difference between plain sautéed chicken breast and chicken cordon bleu. Certain scents, colors, tastes, and images are combined in specific ways because they communicate something important. These symbols will alter your state of consciousness, your perception of yourself, and the way the world relates to you. It's an act of self-care to set aside special time for that.

So, take the time to gather your herbs and light all the candles you want, lovelies. These spells were collected and created with the intention to honor, love, respect, and care for the perfect, divine creature that you are.

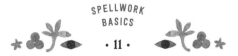

How to Use
This Book

Each spell in this book includes a note on timing and a list of things you will need. Use the following general steps to frame your spellwork as you see fit.

In the back of this book, you will find lists of magical correspondences, places to purchase magical supplies, and useful information about astrology, symbols, and divination. The ingredient lists for these spells are created because they work together in a certain way; however, you can use the information in the back of the book to make substitutions if need be. This first section and the appendix in the back can give you some context and information to work with as you find your own magic.

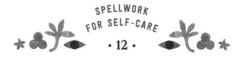

Advance Preparation

WARDING

Wards are magical protections for your space, sort of like magical walls. When you ward your space, you are creating a boundary for your safety. Do this once in your living space (or wherever you are practicing magic), and then periodically "feed" your wards using the instructions at the end of this elemental warding ritual.

YOU WILL NEED:

A bell
A small bowl of salt water
Matches or a lighter
A bundle of sage

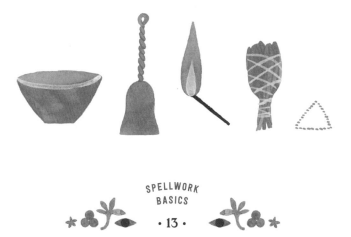

Determine where the boundaries of your wards will be. It's important to respect others' space. Ask family members or roommates if you can ward the home. (If you don't want to ask, or if anyone is uncomfortable with this, just ward your own bedroom or the space right around your bed.) Physically clean that space, clearing it of all clutter and dust.

Walk through every room in the space you are warding, ringing your bell loudly to clear the energy.

Starting in the eastern corner of your space, take the bowl of salt water and sprinkle some along the perimeter of your wards, using your fingers. As you do so, say:

> By water and salt, I ward thee:
> Guard this space from all ill will
> and all those who wish me/us harm.

Imagine that your space is guarded by tall cliffs with waterfalls pouring over them. Pass the salt water over windows and doors twice for more protection.

Light the sage and, starting in the east, waft the smoke along the perimeter of your wards. As you do so, say:

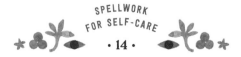

By fire and air, I ward thee:
Guard this space from all ill will
and all those who wish me/us harm.

Imagine your space is now guarded by fierce winds and leaping flames. Pass the sage over windows and doors twice for more protection.

Feed your wards periodically by imagining these boundaries around your space. One way to do this is to imagine light coming from the palms of your hands and directing it to the boundaries of your wards, strengthening the barrier you've already created.

Materials and Timing

The lunar phase and day of the week guidelines in each spell will help you to plan the right time for your working. Timing the spell this way optimizes your magic, but you can certainly choose your own timing as it suits you. Before the time arrives, gather the materials you need. There is also room for creativity in the preparation of your ritual space. You can add objects, lighting, colors, music, and clothing to create an atmosphere that enhances your spellwork.

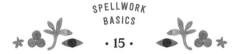

ALTARS

A working altar is useful for spellwork, and some of the spells in this book call for an altar. This is a sacred space that can be as small as a bookshelf dedicated to your spirituality or as large as a coffee table. Items usually found on the altars of magical practitioners include statues or images of deities or saints, items involved in current workings, candles, incense, an offering bowl, and/or ritual tools. Use the appendix in the back of the book to uncover the inherent symbolism in the items you might choose to put on your altar.

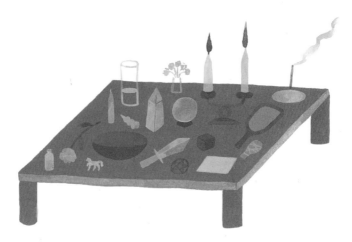

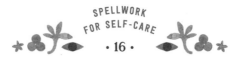

TOOLS

The spells in this book do not require ritual tools. In Wicca, tools used include the athame, wand, chalice, and pentacle. Other practitioners may also use an athame or wand to direct their energy. If you decide to work with one or more of these tools, you should consecrate each item before the first use. Use this consecration when spells call for other items to be consecrated as well.

CONSECRATION

Mix some salt with water and sprinkle this on the item, saying:

> I consecrate this _____ with the
> power of Water and Earth.

Light incense and hold the item in the smoke. Say:

> I consecrate this _____ with the
> power of Fire and Air.
> This _____ is now consecrated,
> bound to aid me in my magical endeavors.

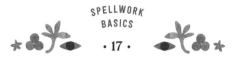

Steps to Spellwork

CLEARING

Having already warded your living area, physically clean the space where you will be performing your spellwork. Stand in the center of that space. Imagine that it is the center of the entire universe. Say:

> *Hekas, Hekas, este bebeloi*
> **(Far, far be removed the profane)**

After speaking these words, use your hands to physically clear the space around you. Arms outstretched with palms facing downward, deliberately push your hands away from each other, as if to sweep through the air around you. Imagine you are physically pushing away any unwanted energy.

According to the Order of the Golden Dawn, these banishing words come from the ancient Eleusinian Mysteries. There are many other clearing rituals. Research and find one that works well for you.

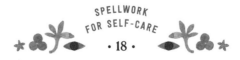

GROUNDING

Before performing spellwork, it's important to clear your mind and ground your energy. To do magic successfully, you need to be fully present. The four-cycle breath is one easy meditation technique for beginners:

Find a comfortable seated position and close your eyes. Take a deep breath in, counting to four. Hold that breath for four counts. Let it out for four counts. Hold your breath for four counts. If you find your mind wandering, simply bring it back, continuing to count your breath. Repeat this cycle until you feel grounded and ready to proceed.

Develop an ongoing meditation practice as part of your daily routine to enhance your spellwork, your spiritual journey, and your life in general. There are a number of apps, including Headspace and Calm, that provide guided meditations to help you develop your own practice.

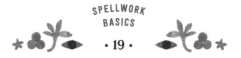

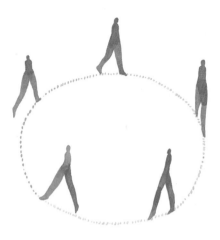

CASTING CIRCLE

Next, create an energetic boundary around your spellworking space. Make room for an invisible circle of about five to six feet in diameter around your materials. Then, walk the perimeter of the circle, starting on the east side of the room and moving clockwise. Say:

> I cast this circle with mind and heart
> A world within and a world apart

These circle-casting words come from the Feri tradition of witchcraft. Continue to research and experiment with different ways of casting circle.

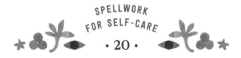

INVOKING SPIRITS

It's common to invite some manifestation of the four directions (North, South, East, and West) to your circle. This is often referred to as "calling the quarters."

Move around the room to face each direction
as you call them, saying:

Spirits of the East, powers of Air, I invite you to join my circle. Hail and welcome!

Spirits of the South, powers of Fire, I invite you to join my circle. Hail and welcome!

Spirits of the West, powers of Water, I invite you to join my circle. Hail and welcome!

Spirits of the North, powers of Earth, I invite you to join my circle. Hail and welcome!

Next, invoke any deities or spirits you intend to work with. You can use the same language you used to call the quarters:

I invite you to join my circle.
Hail and welcome!

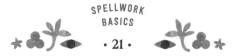

The Work

Once you have cast your circle, called the quarters, and invoked any spirits or deities, you are ready to do your spellwork. This is often called "the work" of the ritual.

DECASTING CIRCLE

After your spellwork is done, it's time to thank all spirits and deities present and to decast your circle. This is also called "spiraling out," because you begin with the last invocation and move backward through the steps you took to cast the circle.

Thank any additional deities or spirits you invited, in the reverse order in which you invited them. Then thank the quarters, in the reverse direction from which you called them.

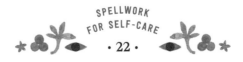

Starting in the North this time, say:

Spirits of the North, powers of Earth, thank you for joining my circle. Hail and farewell!

Continue with the West:

Spirits of the West, powers of Water, thank you for joining my circle. Hail and farewell!

Move to the South and say:

Spirits of the South, powers of Fire, thank you for joining my circle. Hail and farewell!

Ending in the East, say:

Spirits of the East, powers of Air, thank you for joining my circle. Hail and farewell!

Walk around the perimeter of your circle counterclockwise, from north to east, visualizing the boundary disappearing. Your circle has now been opened.

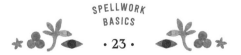

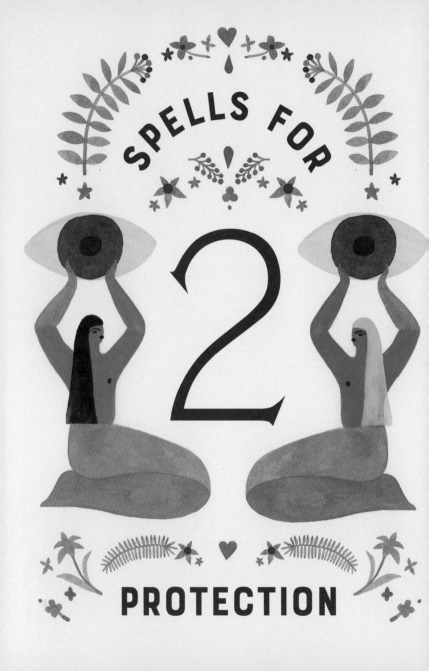

SPELLS FOR

2

PROTECTION

INVOKE A
GUARDIAN

Local spirits and guardians are some of the best
sources of protection for your home. The Romans
called the guardian spirits of the home *Lares*.
Families kept statues of the *Lar* of the home and
left offerings by the hearth to ensure blessings on
the household and all of its inhabitants.

TIMING:
Any time

YOU WILL NEED:

A small offering for the *Lar* of your home, like a slice
of pound cake or some grapes

Optional: incense

Place your offering by the fireplace in your home. If you do not
have a fireplace, the kitchen (especially the stove) serves as the
modern-day hearth. Bless the offering by making the symbol of
manifestation (a triangle with your thumbs and index fingers).

· spell continues ·

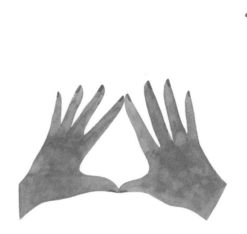

Say:

> **I bless this offering by the power of**
> **Air, Fire, Water, and Earth.**

Light the incense and/or set out your offering in a pretty plate or bowl. Say:

> **Lar, guardian of this place our home,**
> **We honor and welcome you**
> **as a member of our family.**
> **Enjoy this offering as a token of thanks**
> **For the protection and luck you**
> **bring to this household.**

SET PSYCHIC
BOUNDARIES

Maintaining boundaries is essential for self-care.
This means being able to say no when you
don't want to do something and setting psychic
boundaries that keep you from absorbing
too much emotional pain from others. Some
people will drain your energy without even
meaning to. Use this spell to create a light
but powerful barrier between your emotions
and those of others.

TIMING:

Any time

YOU WILL NEED:

A quiet, peaceful place
where you can concentrate

· spell continues ·

Sit in a comfortable position and close your eyes. Take deep breaths in and out, counting to four each time. Focus only on your breathing for ten full breaths. Then, still concentrating on the breath, imagine that you are breathing in positive white light and breathing out any negativity, anxiety, or fear in the form of darkness. Breathe in the white light, letting it fill you. Breathe out the black, watching it dissipate into nothing as soon as it leaves your body.

Once you feel that you have released any lingering anxiety or fear, imagine the white light within you radiating out through the crown of your head. See the light flow around you to surround you entirely in a bubble or shield; every part of your body is protected. Notice how you can move within your shield and it moves with you. Notice how nothing unwanted can pass through the shield of white light. This light came from within you. Let it lift your energy and protect you from low vibrations.

When you see yourself fully surrounded by your shield, open your eyes slowly. This spell will fade over time. Repeat it daily, or when you are preparing to enter situations for which you want a psychic shield.

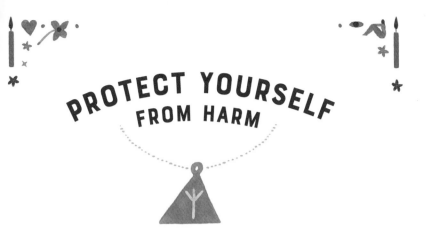

PROTECT YOURSELF
FROM HARM

People have carried good luck charms, amulets, and talismans for centuries. All of these magical objects are used to assist with a specific goal. This one is for protection.

TIMING:

Lunar Phase: Any

Day: Saturday

YOU WILL NEED:

Black polymer clay

A rolling pin

A small carving tool (for example, a metal cuticle pusher)

A cord or chain if you want to wear the talisman as a necklace

· spell continues ·

Think about the feeling of being protected as you make this talisman, channeling feelings of safety into the clay. Roll the clay out until you have a small rectangle about ⅛ inch thick.

Algiz is a Norse guardian rune that wards away harm:

ᛉ

Use the carving tool to etch Algiz into the talisman.

If you plan to wear it on a string as a necklace, make a hole at the top of your talisman. Bake the talisman according to the directions on the package of clay.

Once the talisman has baked and cooled, consecrate it (see page 17) and bless it with these words:

> Baked in fire, cooled by air
> I carved this rune to bless and wear.
> A shield, a sword, a talisman
> Algiz, protect me wherever I am.

TRAVEL SAFELY
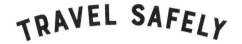

Mojo bags, also known as gris-gris bags, conjure hands, or lucky hands, come from the African-American hoodoo tradition. This is a spell to carry with you for safety while you travel.

TIMING:

Lunar Phase: Waxing Moon or Full Moon

Day: Thursday

YOU WILL NEED:

A slip of paper and a pen

A small blue bag with a drawstring closure

A piece of amethyst

A pinch of mugwort

A pinch of comfrey*

A pinch of fennel seeds

*Comfrey is not safe to ingest.

· spell continues ·

Setting an intention for safe travel, protection, and good fortune, draw the sigil of Jupiter on the paper:

2

Place the paper inside the drawstring bag. Still concentrating on the protection, safety, and luck this bag will bring you, add the amethyst and the herbs. Close and consecrate the bag (see page 17). Say:

> I carry you for luck and safety.
> Stone and herb and sigil drawn,
> In travels near and far embrace me.
> I call you into life with song.

Carry this bag with you or keep it in your car for safe travels.

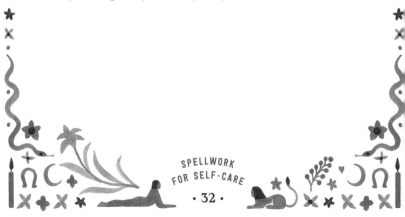

RENEW YOUR
LUCK

Using cleansing and protective magic regularly will help maintain your personal and household safety. Sometimes, however, people get stuck. When the going gets tough—as it inevitably will sometimes—we reach a point where we need a stronger spell to release negativity and move forward. This spell washes away bad luck, leaving you renewed and ready for a fresh start.

TIMING:

Lunar Phase: Waning Crescent Moon

Day: Monday

YOU WILL NEED:

A small saucepan

¼ ounce of dried hyssop

¼ ounce of dried agrimony

A handful of Dead Sea salt

A small jar or bottle

· spell continues ·

Fill the saucepan with water and bring it to a boil. Once the water is boiling, pour in the hyssop and agrimony, remove the pan from the heat and leave the herbs to steep. Once you decide that the water is sufficiently infused with the herbs, strain it and bring it into the bathroom with you.

Run hot water for your bath. Add the Dead Sea salt, along with the herb-infused water, to the bathwater. As you do so, set an intention to wash away all negative energy that has been keeping you stuck. Pour some of the water over your head and soak in the bath.

Before you drain the tub, put some of the bathwater in your jar or bottle. While you watch the water drain, visualize your troubles going down the drain along with it.

After you get dressed, take the bottle of water to a crossroads away from your home and dump it out. Leaving the water at a crossroads disperses the negative energy magically, taking it out of your life so you can move on.

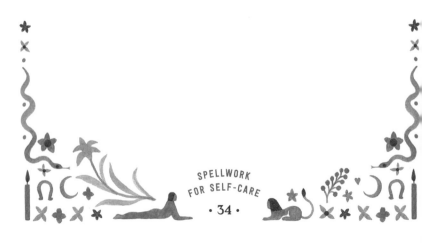

OPEN THE ROAD

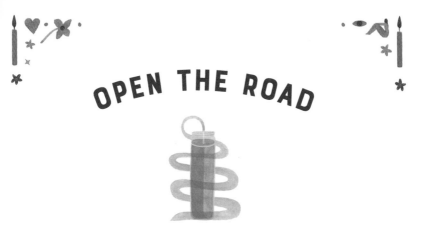

Abre camino means "open road." This plant is commonly found in tropical and semi-tropical climates. Its use in magic and religious rituals comes mostly from the Afro-Cuban religion Santeria. Use this all-purpose spell when you are not sure where you're headed or when you need to remove obstacles from your path.

TIMING:

Lunar Phase: Waning Moon

Day: Thursday

YOU WILL NEED:

A green 7-day candle in a glass jar

Abre camino oil

· spell continues ·

Choose an intention as you take the candle out of its glass container. You might be feeling stuck in a job search and want to open the road to success, or you might be tired of being single and want more opportunities to meet people, so you open the road to love.

Put some of the abre camino oil on your fingers and rub it on the candle from bottom to top, concentrating on your intention to open the way. Say:

**Remove all obstacles
and open my roads to _____.**

If your aim is not specific, you can cover all your bases with "health, love, money, and luck."

Put the candle back in the glass and light it. Stare into the flame and visualize the road opening to your desired path.

This spell requires the candle to burn over a period of seven days. Do not leave burning candles unattended. Snuff the candle when you go to bed or leave the house and relight it with the same intention when you return.

Once the candle has burned down, you can read any images that appear in the wax or smoke residue left on the glass for signs about your working.

RELEASE FEAR

Releasing old fears is a crucial step to
personal growth and empowerment. Use this
spell to empower yourself to move forward.

TIMING:

Lunar Phase: Waning Moon

Day: Saturday

YOU WILL NEED:

A slip of paper and a pen

A small cauldron or bowl for burning

Matches or a lighter

A small trowel

Do this spell outside somewhere that you can safely burn and bury
the paper. Write down what you fear. It might be a fear of failure, of
public speaking, or of being different from others. Put the paper in
your cauldron and burn it, saying:

I burn this fear to be released.

Banish this so I am free.

Bury the ashes of your fear and walk away without looking back.

RELEASE APPROVAL ADDICTION

Like many young womxn, you may constantly worry about what other people think. You may even feel that you cannot make decisions without the approval of others. Take control of your own life by releasing yourself from this anxiety. This is a spell for taking the power of approval out of the hands of others and putting it back in your own hands, where it belongs.

TIMING:

Lunar Phase: New Moon

Day: Any

YOU WILL NEED:

A black crayon

A hard-boiled egg

A mortar and pestle

A bowl of water and a clean towel

Think about a recent moment when you were consumed with worry about what others thought of you. What were you afraid of? What did you want people to think? Using the crayon, write a few words that represent your fears on the shell of the egg. Peel the egg and crush the shell into a powder using the mortar and pestle. As you grind the eggshell, imagine the people whose approval you desire stepping back, the power fading from them and coming back to you.

Now, place the peeled egg in the bowl of water to cleanse it of this negativity. Imagine the egg filling with all of your thoughts of self-approval, confidence, and kind words. Dry the egg carefully with the clean towel and eat it, visualizing these new, positive thoughts filling you from the inside out.

Take your bowl of eggshell powder to a crossroads, and, facing away from the wind, toss it into the air.

As you do so, say:

> Fears of another's secret mind,
> Inner critic's words unkind,
> I release you now, to the four winds blown.
> My approval belongs to me alone.

ACCESS YOUR
STRENGTH

Taking good care of yourself often demands
courage. You have to access your bravery and
overcome your fears to take a risk for love,
to speak up for yourself, or to chase a dream. This
is a spell for accessing the strength that exists
within you. Call on your strength when you need
to do something that scares you.

TIMING:

Lunar Phase: Waxing Moon

Day: Sunday

YOU WILL NEED:

Tarot card: Strength

Water glass

Orange or yellow paper

A black pen

Scissors

Put the Strength card on your altar. Using the glass, trace eight circles on the colored paper and cut them out, so that you have eight disks. You can decorate them to look like the sun or leave them plain.

Think about the times you have accessed your strength before: a time when you were brave, when you overcame an obstacle, or when you stood up for yourself. Write a word (or several) on each disk to represent a time of strength, so that you have eight different reminders of your own power. Arrange the disks in a circle around the Strength card.

Read these words aloud to yourself. Using your finger, draw the infinity symbol (an 8 on its side) on your stomach. Imagine it as golden sunlight imbuing you with the bravery you have demonstrated before. Say:

> **Strength lives in my heart,**
> **Strength lives in my head,**
> **Strength lives in my spirit,**
> **Guiding me always**
> **Like the light of the sun.**

Access this strength to overcome obstacles in your life. You can carry your bravery disks and/or the Strength card with you as talismans.

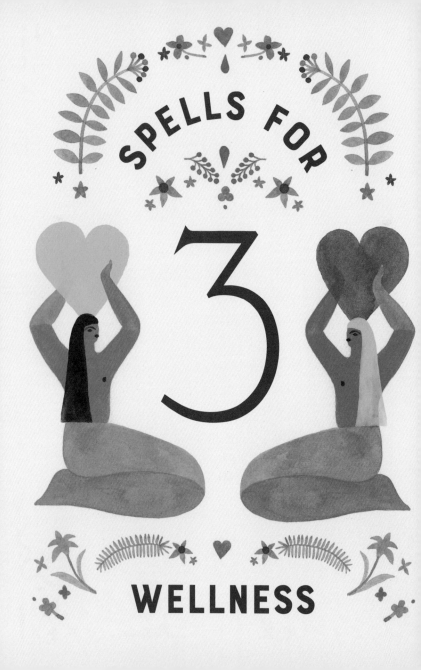

SPELLS FOR

3

WELLNESS

KEEP YOUR FAMILY
HEALTHY

Health is an essential part of prosperity.
Juniper, which has been used to
ward off sickness since ancient times,
has many magical uses, particularly for
protection and prosperity magic.
This potent spell will keep you and
your family well.

TIMING:

Lunar Phase: Waxing Moon or Full Moon

Day: Monday or Thursday

YOU WILL NEED:

Juniper incense*

A blue ribbon or cord made of natural materials,
at least 12 inches long

*Juniper is unsafe for pregnancy. Don't use juniper incense if
you are pregnant or trying to become pregnant. Please see the
list of possible substitutions on page 117.

· spell continues ·

Cast this spell at night, under the moon.

Light the incense. Take your ribbon or cord and say:

> ### I call upon the powers that be
> ### To bring good health to my family.

Pass the cord through the smoke of the lighted juniper incense to purify and imbue it with strength and protection. Concentrate on good health as you begin to tie a series of knots. You will be tying knots in this order:

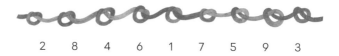

2   8   4   6   1   7   5   9   3

Tie the first knot in the middle of the cord and say:

> ### By the knot of one, the spell has begun.

Tie a knot on the left-hand end of the cord and say:

> ### By the knot of two, it will come true.

Tie a knot on the right-hand end of the cord, saying:

By the knot of three, so shall it be.

Continue to tie the knots according to the order on the facing page, saying these words:

By the knot of four, it is strengthened more.

By the knot of five, so may it thrive.

By the knot of six, this spell is fixed.

By the knot of seven, be it powered by the heavens.

By the knot of eight, guide the hand of fate.

By the knot of nine, the thing is mine.

So mote it be.

Pass the knotted cord through the smoke of the lighted juniper incense to seal the spell. Hang the cord near a doorway or window to keep your family in good health.

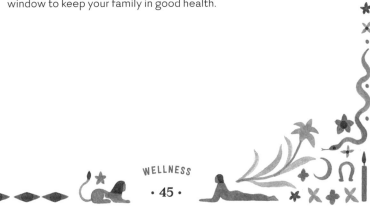

LOVE YOURSELF

This self-love bath will help you see yourself—and treat yourself—as the radiant being you are. Self-love is where self-care begins. Soak in this bath as a way to care for yourself, ensuring that you can access all of your magic.

TIMING:

Lunar Phase: Waxing Moon or Full Moon

Day: Friday

YOU WILL NEED:

Essential oil of rose

Rose petals

One or more pieces of rose quartz

A self-love mantra

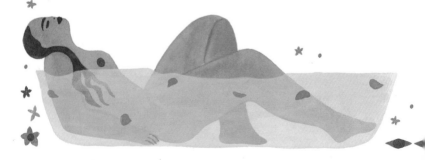

Run hot water for your bath and add a few drops of the essential oil. As you do so, say:

Into this water I pour love,
Let it flow from within me, around, and above.

Repeat three times, putting a little more oil into the bathwater each time. Skim your hand across the water to distribute the scent. Add rose petals and rose quartz, and concentrate on the love that is flowing through the water.

Once you are in the bath, savor the soothing heat of the water, the pleasing scent, and the beauty that surrounds you. You have given this to yourself because you're inherently worthy of pleasure. Repeat your chosen mantra five times as you soak in the bath. Soak up all of the love you have poured into the water.

When you're ready, drain the bath, visualizing all of your self-criticism flowing out of you and away with the water, down the drain. Visualize yourself surrounded in a radiant green light. Say:

By the power of Venus,
I have bathed myself in love.
Love flows from within me, around, and above.
So mote it be.

RELEASE
A BAD HABIT

Developing the discipline to break
bad habits is part of caring for yourself.
Use this spell to commit to letting go
of a procrastination habit, a junk food
addiction, or any other impediment
to your self-care. It will give you some
magical support to finally move on.

TIMING:

Lunar Phase: Waning Moon

Day: Any

YOU WILL NEED:

A slip of paper and a pen

A small cauldron or bowl that is safe for
burning

Matches or a lighter

Write the habit you want to release on the piece of paper. Fold it in half, with the open side facing away from you, and then fold it in half again, still folding it away from you. Say:

**Break the cycle, start anew,
Let fire burn this habit through.**

Put the paper in the cauldron or bowl and set it on fire. Visualize your bad habit disappearing with the smoke.

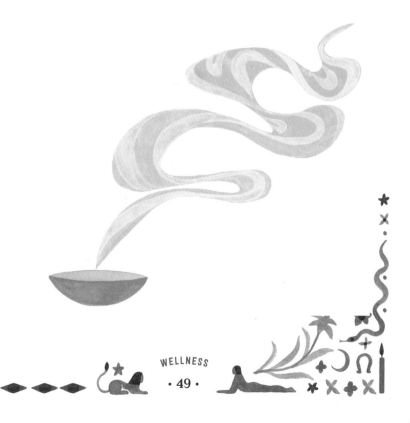

INCREASE YOUR VITALITY

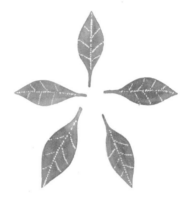

A petition is essentially a prayer to a
spirit or deity for something you want.
If you're feeling low, getting over a
cold, or you're generally drained, this
spell is a good pick-me-up.

TIMING:

Lunar Phase: Waxing Moon

Day: Tuesday

YOU WILL NEED:

A slip of paper and a pen

A small plate

5 fresh basil leaves

A red candle

On the paper, write your name four times. In an unbroken circle around the edges, write the word *vitality*, repeating it until the circle is closed. As you do this, picture yourself healthy, happy, and thriving. This is your petition.

Place the plate on your altar with the paper on top. Arrange your basil leaves around the paper in the shape of a pentagram (a five-pointed star). Place the candle on top of the paper. Say:

> By this sweet basil and flame of red,
> I ask to renew my vitality.
> Give me energy for the days ahead
> that I may be strong and free.

Light the candle. Let it burn down so that the wax covers the petition. Leave this on your altar until the spell is done.

SYNC YOUR CYCLE
WITH THE MOON

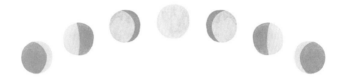

For those who menstruate, your cycle provides
an opportunity for mindfulness and self-care
when synced with the earth's natural cycles.
Typically, a menstrual cycle lasts approximately
twenty-eight days, which is just as long as it
takes for the moon to grow from new to full and
back again. Tracking your personal cycle
in conjunction with the moon's phases will help
you get in touch with your body in a new
and natural way.

YOU WILL NEED:

2 quarts of water

8 teaspoons of dried red raspberry
leaves, or 8 red raspberry leaf tea bags

A covered carafe

A blank calendar with new, full,
and quarter moons listed

For this spell, you'll make a big batch of tea. (Alternatively, you can brew yourself one bag of tea each day.) While you heat the water in a pot on the stove, place your hands over the raspberry leaves or tea bags and say:

> I bless these leaves of raspberry
> That they may bring me healing peace.
> As I brew this tonic tea
> I am one with the rhythm of land, sky, and sea.

Once the water has come to a boil, place your leaves or tea bags in the water, remove the pot from the heat, and let it steep for ten to fifteen minutes. Then strain the tea into your carafe. Pour yourself a cup.

· spell continues ·

As you sip your tea, take a look at your calendar. Mark today, the first day of your cycle, with the number 1. Make some notes on the calendar about how you feel. Notice where the moon is in her cycle.* Visualize your own energy waxing and waning along with the moon.

Store your carafe of tea in the refrigerator. Drink a small cup each day, say the spell words, and record observations about your cycle for the next twenty-eight days (or until your next period). You may need to brew another batch of tea.

You can use your observations of your own cycle and the moon's to plan your days as your energy waxes and wanes.

Raspberry leaf tea balances your hormones, reduces acne associated with your period, eases the flow of menstrual blood, and relieves cramping by relaxing and strengthening your uterine walls.

*If the date is between the new and full moon, the moon is waxing. If the date is between the full moon and the next new moon, the moon is waning.

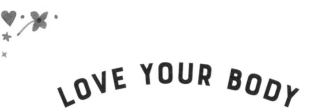

LOVE YOUR BODY

Self-love includes accepting your body for
all of its beauty *and* its imperfections. Use
this ritual to help yourself feel good about
who you are, inside and out.

TIMING:

Lunar Phase: Any

Day: Friday

YOU WILL NEED:

A piece of rose quartz

A full-length mirror

A journal and a pen

Stand in front of a full-length mirror, taking the time to look at
every part of yourself from the top of your head to the tips
of your toes. Notice the thoughts that arise as you observe your
own image. Are you critical of certain parts of yourself? Where
do you think that comes from? Take notice of your positive
thoughts about yourself, too.

· spell continues ·

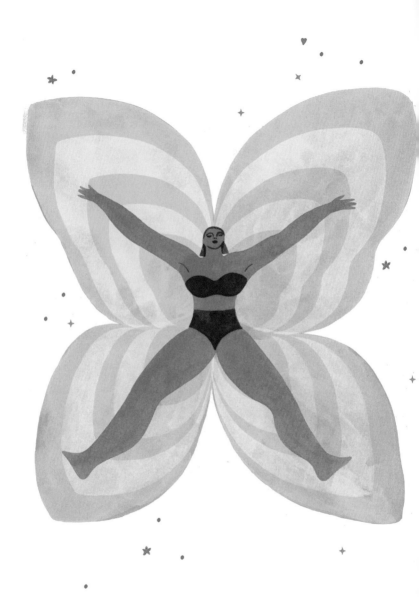

Once you become aware of the thoughts you have about your body, take some time to reframe any negative thoughts. If your thought is "I hate my big thighs," find a new way to look at that part of yourself. You don't have to affirm something, like "I love my thighs," if you don't feel that it's true right now. Lying to yourself will not be effective. Just find something true that feels better than the negative thought. For example, "My strong, sturdy legs get me everywhere" is a true statement with a much more positive vibration. Focusing on what your body does for you helps take some emphasis off your appearance.

In your journal, make a list of seven parts of your body and write a positive or reframed thought next to each one. Here are some examples:

1 • Arms: My arms are nice and tan right now.

2 • Hands: My hands play the piano with grace.

3 • Eyes: I have beautiful, mysterious eyes.

Now, take the rose quartz and touch it to each part of your body on the list, one by one. Read your positive statements out loud to yourself and feel the change in your body as you treat yourself with gentle kindness. Repeat this once a day for seven days.

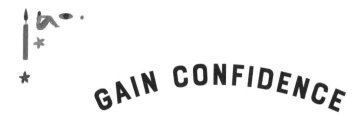

GAIN CONFIDENCE

You were born to radiate your incandescent light. If you're not used to it, however, shining can be scary! Perform this spell when you need the confidence to shine from within.

TIMING:

Lunar Phase: Waxing Moon
or Full Moon

Day: Sunday

YOU WILL NEED:

A small carving tool (for example,
a metal cuticle pusher)

A yellow candle

An orange

Carve your name along with a glyph of the sun into the candle. Add any other carvings that speak to you of confidence, sunshine, happiness, and success. Consult pages 115, 121, and 122 for ideas.

Peel the orange and split it into segments. Arrange them around the candle on your altar. As you light the candle, say:

> As I light this candle flame
> Let the light within me grow.
> Courage and confidence is my aim,
> Fire within me shine and glow.

Enjoy the orange pieces as you watch the candle flicker. Visualize each segment of orange as a piece of the sun that is lighting you up from the inside. Leave one or two segments on the altar as an offering. Respectfully dispose of these outside the next day.

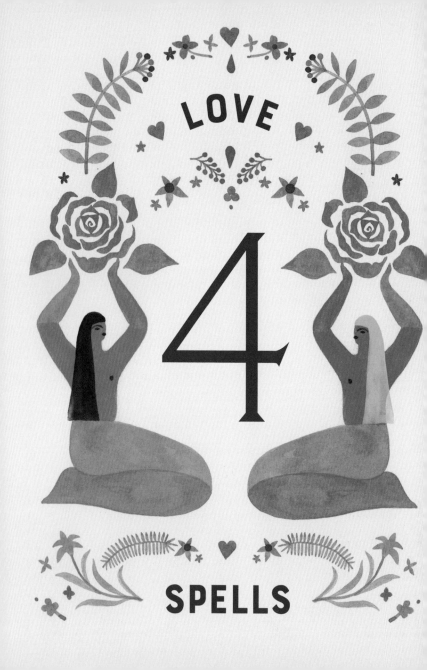

SPREAD
GOODWILL

Spells can be baked or brewed into everyday food and drink with a little know-how and conscious intention. Sugar is frequently used in spells to sweeten relations between people, and lavender promotes peace. These lavender-scented sugar cookies will spread goodwill to friends, family, and neighbors who enjoy their sweet taste.

TIMING:

Any time

YOU WILL NEED:

Ingredients for your favorite
basic sugar cookie recipe

1½ teaspoons of dried lavender buds
per 1 dozen cookies

Vanilla frosting

Optional: decorative frosting tube

· spell continues ·

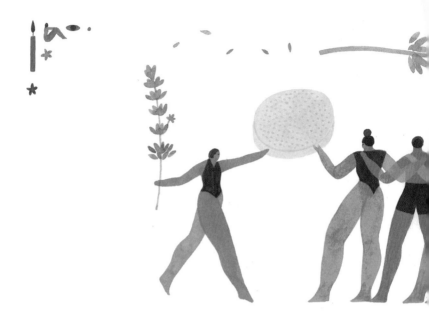

The night before you plan to bake your cookies, measure out the sugar for your chosen recipe. Combine the lavender buds with the sugar in a medium-size bowl and place the bowl in an east-facing window to let the sun's first rays hit it at dawn. The lavender will perfume the sugar, enhancing the flavor of the cookies.

When you're ready to bake, arrange your ingredients on the counter. Take several deep breaths. Visualize spending time with a friend you love. Feel the happiness that you experience when you're with that friend. Set an intention to let those same feelings of love, happiness, and friendship flow through you into the cookies that you bake.

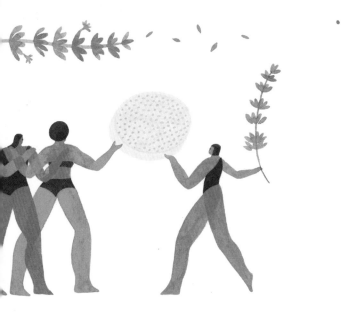

As you blend the ingredients together to form the dough, say:

> **May all who taste this fragrant cookie**
> **Enjoy friendship, peace, and harmony.**

Bake the cookies as directed in the recipe, using your lavender sugar. Frost the cookies once they cool. If you want to get really fancy, you can decorate them with magical symbols, such as a heart shape or the glyph of Venus (see page 115) to symbolize good relationships.

Share the cookies with family members, neighbors, classmates, and anyone else with whom you want to spread goodwill!

BRING HARMONY TO YOUR HOUSEHOLD

Honey jar spells are often used to sweeten relationships with other people, combining the sweetness of sugar with herbs intended to promote positivity. Use this spell to create a peaceful environment in your home, or to pacify a situation between household members if things have been less than harmonious.

TIMING:

Lunar Phase: Waxing Moon or Full Moon

Day: Sunday, Monday, Wednesday, Thursday, or Friday

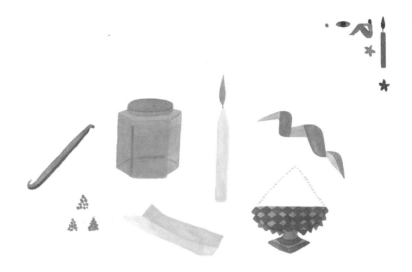

YOU WILL NEED:

A clean glass jar with a lid

Sugar

A slip of paper and a pen

A pinch of thyme

A pinch of sage

A pinch of ground cloves

A pinch of orange zest

1 whole vanilla bean

A small white candle

· spell continues ·

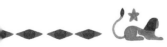

LOVE

Choose a name for your household. If your family's last name is Smith, for example, "The Smith Family" works just fine. You can also invent a household name to use in protective magic.

Fill your jar almost full with sugar, leaving some room for the other ingredients. Write the name of your household four times on the slip of paper. Without letting the pen leave the paper, write the word *harmony* around the edges, repeating it until you've created a circle around your household name.

Fold the paper in half toward you, and say:

> I conjure peace and harmony.
> By sugar sweet, three herbs, and fruit,
> Protect our home and family.

Continue folding the paper toward you until you can't fold it any more.

Take a taste of the sugar, visualizing the sweetness of harmony in your home. Then bury the paper in the jar so that you can no longer see it. Add the thyme, sage, ground cloves, and orange zest. Add the vanilla bean and close the jar. Put the candle on top of the lid, light it, and let it burn down to seal the jar with its wax.

Keep your honey jar on your altar and periodically burn a new candle on it to renew the spell.

FIND YOUR
GLAMOUR

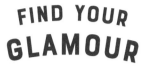

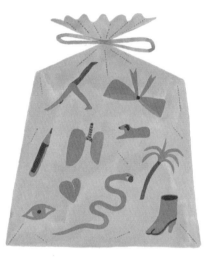

True glamour is just the carefully calibrated projection of what makes you special. It is not about imitation. It is embracing your magnetic otherness and using it to draw people to you. Use this spell to find your own special glamour.

· spell continues ·

LOVE

YOU WILL NEED:

A small drawstring bag,
preferably decorated with a design you like

Collect small beautiful things that represent you. These could include beads, scraps of fabric from old clothes, photographs, pictures from magazines, poems, feathers, shells, and/or stones. Edit your collection until it feels right to you. Put all of these things in your bag. Say:

> By this bag of baubles found
> Let my glamour come to me.
> Magnetic aura thus surround
> An air of subtle mystery.

Carry this bag with you until you feel that the glamour has become part of your aura, and then put it somewhere for safekeeping.

Note: This spell is inspired by one of Deborah Castellano's Esoteric Experiments in her book, *Glamour Magic: The Witchcraft Revolution to Get What You Want.*

MAKE NEW
FRIENDS

Good friends support each other, trust
each other, and enjoy each other's company.
Building healthy friendships is another
important aspect of self-care. Use this spell
to call new friends into your life.

TIMING:

Lunar Phase: Waxing Moon

Day: Friday

YOU WILL NEED:

Fresh spring water

3 cups

Tarot card: Three of Cups

Clear a space on a table or countertop and place the three cups
in a row next to each other. Fill each cup a quarter of the way
full with water. Place the tarot card, face up, in front of the cups.
Most tarot decks feature three figures holding their cups aloft

· spell continues ·

in celebration on this card. Imagine you are one of the three figures on the card and the other two are new friends.

Visualize your little party in a place where you would want to spend time with your friends: Picture your trio doing something you enjoy, like going out to eat, skiing, dancing, or swapping secrets late at night. Hold this image in your mind. Say:

> I call to my kindred spirits
> By the light of my north star.
> My social life is growing
> With friends from near and far.

Pick up the cup on the left. Pour that water into the middle cup, then back into the left-hand cup, and finally back into the middle cup. As you do so, say:

> I give to my friends
> And they give to me
> By the power of three.
> So mote it be.

Repeat this with the cup on the right. Say these spell words one more time and then drink from the middle cup. Keep the Three of Cups card on your altar or under your pillow until you meet a new friend.

IMPROVE COMMUNICATION

Mercury is the planet of communication, and fennel is associated with the powers of speech. Good communication is the cornerstone of any good relationship. Do this spell to ensure that you communicate well with the people you love.

TIMING:

Lunar Phase: Waxing Moon

Day: Wednesday

YOU WILL NEED:

Fennel seeds

· spell continues ·

Using the fennel seeds, draw the glyph of Mercury (see page 115) outside on the ground. Say:

Powers of speech and thoughts so clear,
Help me understand another.
I listen well; when I speak they hear,
We communicate easily with each other.

Leave this glyph outside for twenty-four hours. You could either plant the fennel seeds afterward or let the birds and other animals take the seeds as an offering.

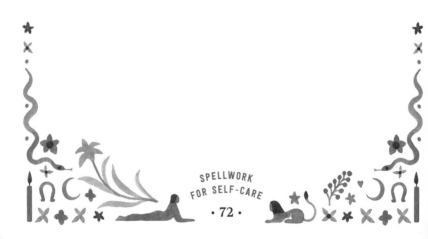

RELEASE A
PAST LOVE

Breakups are emotional and the healing process is different for everyone. Even when you are ready to move on from someone, you may find it difficult to truly release an old relationship. This spell cuts the etheric cords that tied you to your past love, freeing your energy so that you can heal and grow.

TIMING:

Lunar Phase: Waning Moon

Day: Saturday

YOU WILL NEED:

A photo of you and the other person, or 2 scraps of paper

Scissors

A 9-inch length of cord, yarn, or thread

· spell continues ·

LOVE

Taking the photo of the two of you together, cut it in half so that you're split apart. If you have chosen to use two scraps of paper instead, write your name on one piece and your past love's name on the other piece. Roll each photo or piece of paper into a cylinder and tie them up in opposite ends of the cord. As you tie the knots, think about the ties you still have to this person. You have a set of invisible cords that run between you, connecting you energetically. The cord that ties your photos together represents all of those etheric cords.

When you are ready, cut the cord. See the etheric cords that connected you as severed. Recognize that your energy is no longer flowing to this other person. You are released from this burden. You can begin to heal. Bury each photo or paper, with the piece of cord still attached, in separate places.

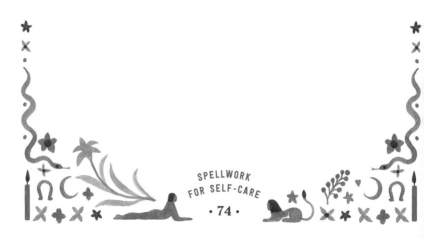

ATTRACT ROMANCE

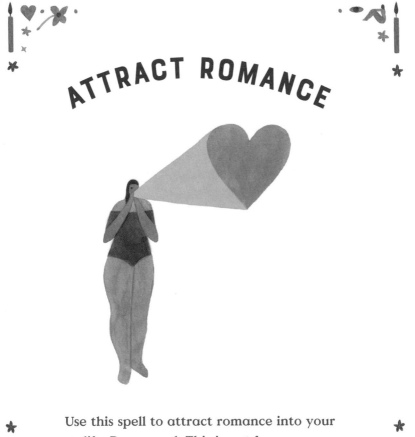

Use this spell to attract romance into your
life. Be warned: This is not for use on
a specific person. This is a spell to attract
the *right* relationship. You may not have
met your future love yet!

· spell continues ·

YOU WILL NEED:

A slip of paper and a pen

A red candle

A red ribbon, string, or piece of yarn

On the slip of paper, write down all of the qualities you would like to have in a partner. Use general terms to describe what you want, because you don't always know what wonderful things lie in store for you. For example, if creativity is important to you, instead of writing "plays guitar," add "creative" to your list.

Next, write about the kind of relationship you want to have with this person. When you're done envisioning your future romance, put the paper under your red candle. Light the candle and say:

> **Bring me my love, right and true.**
> **I open up my heart to you.**

Let the candle burn down. Roll up the paper with the wax or any of the candle that is left, and tie it with the red ribbon. Leave it on your altar or under your pillow until a new romance begins.

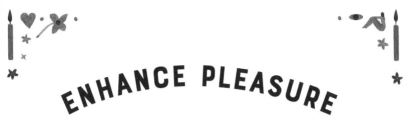

ENHANCE PLEASURE

A major part of self-care is acknowledging and enhancing your pleasure! Use this spell if you're sexually active and you want to increase your pleasure during sex or masturbation. If you are partnered, talk to your partner about what you want in bed. While there is no magic like good communication in a relationship, this chocolate pleasure potion is pretty good, too, combining several aphrodisiacs to maximize your orgasm.

Historically, the female orgasm has been treated by the patriarchy as unimportant, unhealthy, and even nonexistent. Men orgasm more than women, a phenomenon scientists have termed the "orgasm gap." In a study conducted by scientists at Chapman University in California, 95 percent of the heterosexual men reported that they usually-to-always orgasm during sex, compared to 65 percent of the heterosexual women.

· spell continues ·

LOVE

YOU WILL NEED:

2 tablespoons unsweetened cocoa powder

¼ cup of sugar

¼ cup of hot water

2 cups of milk

½ teaspoon of vanilla extract

½ teaspoon of ground cinnamon

Pinch of cayenne pepper

Combine the cocoa powder, sugar, and hot water in a medium saucepan. Over medium heat, stir until the mixture boils. As you stir, say:

Pleasure now, I conjure you with this swirling chocolate brew.

Turn the temperature down and stir in the milk to heat it (but do not let it boil). Take the saucepan off the heat and add the vanilla, cinnamon, and cayenne pepper. Pour the hot chocolate into a mug for yourself (and one for your partner if you're sharing). Drink immediately and climb into bed. Enjoy!

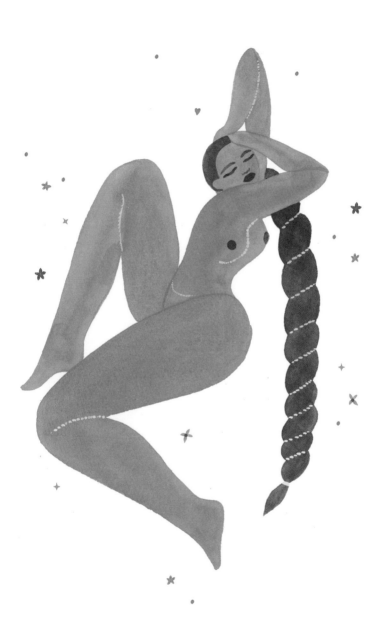

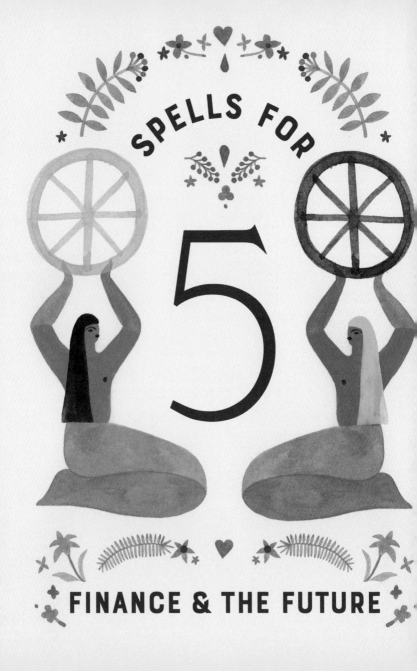

SPELLS FOR

5

FINANCE & THE FUTURE

MANIFEST
ABUNDANCE

This spell calls on Oshun, a goddess of the Yoruba religion, who rules luxury, pleasure, wealth, sexuality, and fertility. She is the goddess of rivers and fresh water, so this working must be completed at a river or stream. Use this spell to ask Oshun for the abundance you desire in your life.

TIMING:

Lunar Phase: Waxing Moon or Full Moon

Day: Friday

YOU WILL NEED:

A round piece of bread (like a dinner roll)

A slip of paper and a pen

Honey

A small yellow candle

· spell continues ·

FINANCE &
THE FUTURE

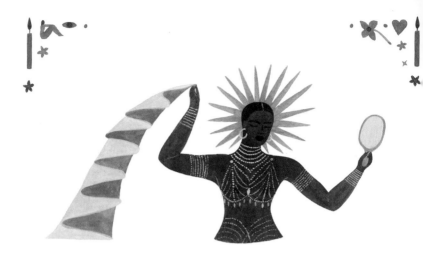

Make a hole in the bread that is just big enough for your candle to sit in, as if it were a candleholder. Write your desires on the paper, fold it, and put it into the hole. Pour some honey on top of the paper. Then place the yellow candle in the hole and light it. While the candle burns down, do something that makes you feel happy, wealthy, and beautiful: eat something tasty, watch a good movie, or paint your nails. When the candle has burned down and covered the bread with melted wax, take this offering to a river or stream. As you toss it into the water, say:

Oshun, goddess of waters sweet,

O beautiful queen of desire,

I give you this honey and bread to eat.

Please help my wishes transpire.

ENVISION YOUR FUTURE

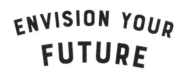

Few things are more powerful than envisioning what you want. Vision boards contain potent magic. The images of your desires will stay in your subconscious and help you to manifest them into reality as time goes on.

TIMING:

Lunar Phase: New Moon

Day: Any

YOU WILL NEED:

Magazines

A piece of poster board or cardboard for your vision board

Scissors

Glue

· spell continues ·

Begin by meditating on how you want to feel in the future—whether it's next year, in five years, or beyond. Do you envision feelings of peace, love, success, ease, excitement, freedom, or something else? Go deep into the meditation to see what you are doing in the future—listen to what it sounds like, enjoy the scents, feel the textures, and taste the fruits of your future happiness.

Following the visualization, flip through some magazines until you find a picture that speaks to you. It doesn't have to make sense or mean anything to you now; it just has to *feel* right. Cut it out and glue it on your vision board. Continue with this process until the board is covered.

When your vision board is complete, hang it somewhere in your home where you will see it but won't be staring at it all the time. Allow yourself to forget about it. Your subconscious will remain aware of your future plans. You'll be amazed at the synchronicities that arise!

The key to a good vision board is to let your subconscious do the driving. It's easy to decide that you want more money and then cut out pictures of cash and fancy cars. But that's actually not as powerful as developing a vision board that follows the thread of your emotions from your present into your future.

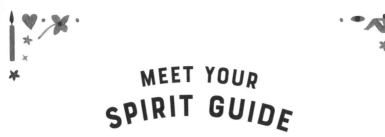

MEET YOUR
SPIRIT GUIDE

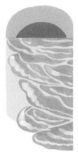

Everyone has a spirit guide—you might even have
several. All you have to do if you want to connect
with yours is reach out. Use this visualization
to begin developing a relationship with your guide.

TIMING:

Any time

YOU WILL NEED:

A white candle

A journal and a pen

· spell continues ·

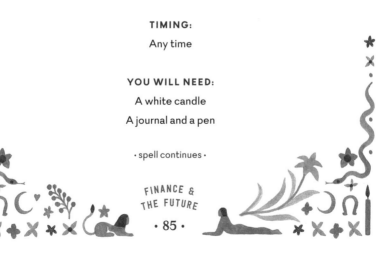

Start with your regular meditation practice to center yourself (see page 19 if you need some guidance). Light the white candle and ask to meet your spirit guide.

Close your eyes and notice the darkness that surrounds you. Envision a pinprick of light, and watch it grow larger until it becomes a doorway. Walk through the doorway and onto a beach. See and hear the water lapping the shore. Wait for your spirit guide to appear. Ask it the following questions:

1 • What is your name?

2 • Do you come only to work with me for my highest good?

3 • What form do you usually take?

4 • Do you have a message for me?

5 • How can I speak with you again?

Accept the first answer that you are given for each question. Pay attention to how you feel around your guide. If the spirit you are talking to is your guide, you will have only good feelings and the answers given will be in your best interests. If you feel uncomfortable at any time, you can leave the beach and come back to your room. Thank your guide once you are finished.

Visualize yourself walking back through the door into the darkness and then become aware of the room around you. Slowly open your eyes. Write about your experience.

SUCCEED IN SCHOOL

Feeding your mind is as important for self-care as feeding your body. Create this special blend of oils to help you focus in school. This spell has you anoint your books with the oil. You can also dab a little bit on your wrists or open the jar to breathe in this scent before you study.

TIMING:

Any time

YOU WILL NEED:

1 part rosemary essential oil

1 part peppermint essential oil

Small glass bottle

· spell continues ·

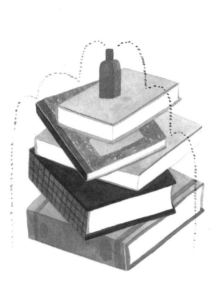

Blend the oils together in the empty bottle, concentrating on your intention to succeed. Place a small drop on your finger and touch it to your schoolbooks one by one to anoint them for success. Say:

**Bless the reader of these books
with disciplined focus and a good memory
for the knowledge within.**

You can adapt this to bless your notebooks, pens, and computer, too. Use this oil blend as an aromatherapy to help you wake up and stay focused in school, or when you're doing homework.

FIND A JOB

Use this incense spell when you
need to find a summer or
part-time job, an internship, or
your first (gulp!) adult job.

TIMING:
Lunar Phase: Waxing Moon or Full Moon
Day: Any

YOU WILL NEED:
A slip of paper and a pen
1 part patchouli incense
1 part birch bark
½ part cedar tips
½ part cinnamon chips
½ part sandalwood incense
A mortar and pestle
Incense burner and charcoal

· spell continues ·

On a slip of paper, write a list of the things you're looking for in a job. As you mix the ingredients for this incense powder with your mortar and pestle, read the items on your list out loud. Put your charcoal in the incense burner, light it, and sprinkle your powder on top. Burn a little bit of this incense every day to attract a new job, especially right before you submit an application or go for an interview.

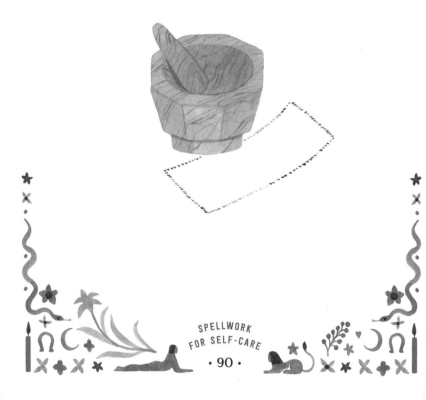

KEEP YOUR
WALLET FULL

A sigil is a magically charged symbol that
expresses the energy of a desire or entity.
This spell calls for you to create your
own prosperity sigil to draw money into
your wallet and keep it there.

TIMING:

Lunar Phase: Waxing Moon or Full Moon

Day: Thursday or Friday

YOU WILL NEED:

A scrap of paper and a ballpoint pen

A small piece of green paper

A silver or gold paint pen or gel pen

· spell continues ·

FINANCE &
THE FUTURE

Before you draw your sigil, make sure your wallet is clean. Take out any expired or unnecessary cards, receipts, or coupons. Organize your bills so they are all face up and neatly pressed. Put excess change in a coin purse or piggy bank. Wipe a damp cloth over your wallet if you need to shine it up a bit. Wealth is attracted to a wallet that looks good!

Write this sentence on your scrap of paper:

MY WALLET IS ALWAYS FULL OF MONEY

Delete all of the vowels and any repeating consonants from this sentence. Rewrite the remaining letters:

MWLTSFN

Use these letters to design your own sigil. Let your creativity guide you (without judgment!) while remaining focused on the intent of the symbol to keep your wallet full of money. Arrange the letters in a circle or make each one a different size, mash them up, turn them upside down, stringing them together in a new sequence to create a symbol of your wealth. By the time you're done with your creation, it shouldn't look like a collection of letters anymore. When you feel that your sigil is complete, carefully copy it onto the green paper with the paint pen. Put it in your wallet, knowing that there will always be money there for you.

BRING PROSPERITY TO YOUR HOUSEHOLD

A floor wash is a hoodoo technique
for cleansing the home of what is not
wanted and drawing prosperity in.

TIMING:

Lunar Phase: Full Moon

Day: Thursday

YOU WILL NEED:

Water in a large pot on the stove

A handful of dried basil

The peel of 1 orange

7 drops of peppermint oil

A bucket and cloth or mop

Bring the water to a boil. Add your dried basil, orange peel, and peppermint oil. Boil this together for about ten minutes. Strain the basil and orange peel out and put the remaining water in your bucket.

Wait for your brew to cool a bit before washing the floor with it. Meditate on the energy of prosperity as you mop.

FINANCE &
THE FUTURE

FIND YOUR
CAREER PATH

When finding a career path, you
have to follow the call from within.
This spell helps you get in touch with
your wild instincts.

TIMING:

Lunar Phase: Waxing Moon or Full Moon

Day: Tuesday

YOU WILL NEED:

A journal and a pen

An image of an animal you feel a
strong connection with, or an offering from that
animal, like a found feather or some fur

An image of this animal's tracks

Consecrate your journal (see page 17). On the first page, paste the image or offering from your chosen animal. Below that, paste or draw an image of the animal's tracks. Write this invocation on the page:

This book reveals the inner call
of the wild [your name]**, the animal**
whose instincts lead her along the path
to career success and happiness.

Say the invocation aloud once you have written it. The journal is now enchanted. Use it only to write about finding your career path, with the following exercises:

1 • Make a list of every activity that you have been totally, happily absorbed in. This is a list of your wild animal tracks.

2 • Make a second list of the attributes your wild tracks activities have in common.

3 • Look around your environment to find alternate activities that relate to the ones on your list. Try one and see where it leads. Track how you feel in your journal as you follow that path.

4 • Research your animal. Write about its symbolic attributes and habits in your journal. What can this animal teach you?

5 • If a trail you are following goes cold (i.e., you feel bored, anxious, or upset while you are engaged in that activity), return to your list of wild tracks and start again. Repeat until you find a path that feels right.

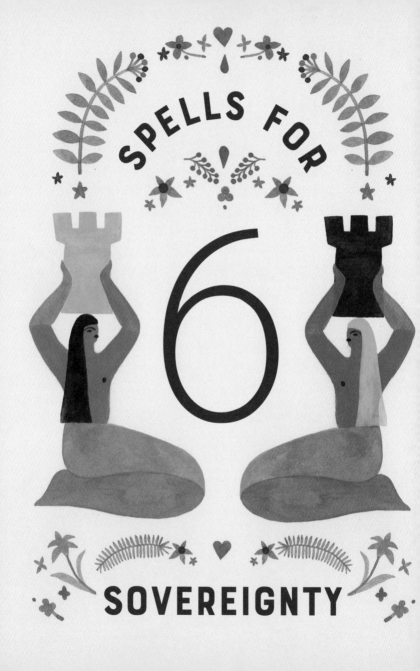

CONNECT WITH YOUR ANCESTORS

Traditions to honor one's ancestors are found
all over the world. It's important to honor
and remember our beloved dead simply
because we love them. In many traditions,
ancestors are also present in our lives
as spirits, able to protect us and help us.

TIMING:

Any time

YOU WILL NEED:

Photos of your recent ancestors (you can
also write their names on nice paper)

Small items that represent them, such as
the feather of a favorite bird or a beloved mug

Fresh flowers

A white candle

A small dish or bowl to hold an offering

· spell continues ·

Set up an ancestor altar using the memorabilia you've collected. Place your photos, commemorative objects, and fresh flowers on a clean shelf, table, or cabinet where you can keep it intact for a long period of time. A wall of family photos over a side table is a perfectly good ancestor altar hiding in plain sight. Just make sure to keep photos of the living separate from photos of the dead.

Light the candle and offer some food or drink that your ancestors liked; fresh spring water and coffee are popular choices. Think of this experience as having your family members over to your house. When they were living, you would offer them something to eat or drink. You can do the same for them even after they have passed.

Gaze at the candle flame and wait for any messages. Look for signs and synchronicity over the next few days. Start talking to your ancestors regularly, through journaling or prayer. Offer them a little something now and then and ask them to watch over you and your family.

Feel free to leave photos or names off the altar if you have ancestors who were not kind people in life. Readers whose families are healing from a generational cycle of abuse, especially, may choose not to include some ancestors. You can also include photos of good friends and respected mentors or elders who have passed away.

REMEMBER
DREAMS

Your dreams are a key to your unconscious
thoughts, and when you work with them often,
they can even contain answers to questions or
information about the future. If you keep a dream
journal regularly, you will remember your dreams
with more clarity and you will start to see patterns.
Use this spell to enhance your dream life.

TIMING:

Any time

YOU WILL NEED:

Dried lavender buds

Dried jasmine flowers

Dried rose petals

Dried orange peel

A white or silver pouch

A journal and a pen

· spell continues ·

Put a little bit of each ingredient into the pouch and shut it tightly. Place this under your pillow. Before you go to sleep each night, say:

> Please guide me through the realm of dreams.
> Show me what I need to see
> And help me remember when I wake.

Record your dreams in your journal each morning when you wake up.

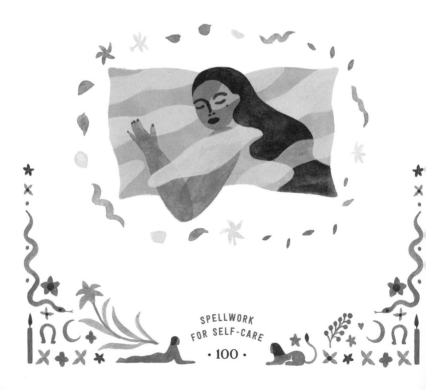

CONNECT WITH THE DIVINE FEMININE

The divine feminine deserves a special place in this book because, as witchy womxn, we are recovering lost arts of healing and magic. Part of self-care for anyone is honoring the feminine within you—that which has been forgotten, degraded, and vilified. There are many pantheons and goddesses whom you might get to know, so this is a ritual for opening the door to connection.

TIMING:

Lunar Phase: Full Moon

Day: Any

YOU WILL NEED:

A natural beeswax candle

A purple cord or ribbon, 9 inches long

Honey

Books and resources on pantheons or goddesses that interest you

· spell continues ·

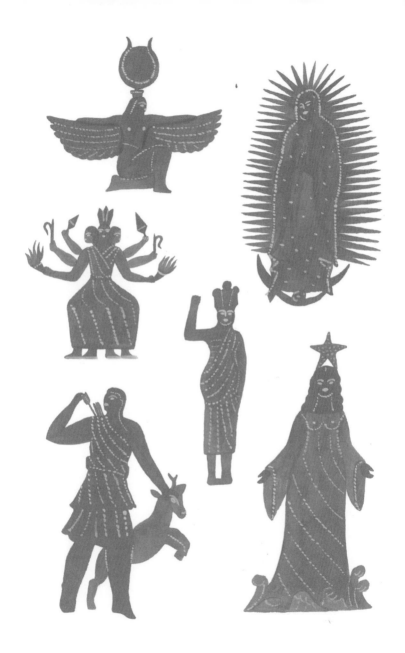

Light the candle. Take the cord between your hands, hold it up to the sky, and say:

> I call on the wisdom of the divine feminine
> Seeking connection and spiritual growth.

Tie nine knots in the cord and wind it around the base of the candle. Pour a bit of honey on the skin between your left thumb and index finger and taste it. Say:

> I taste the sweet honey of the goddess.
> She who is within me,
> She who is all around me,
> Let yourself be known to me.
> So mote it be.

As the candle burns, read about goddesses from different cultures. See if you connect with any one in particular. Watch for signs from her over the next few days. Getting to know a goddess is similar to making friends with a person: you start out slowly, and you may end up being close friends for a long time, or just friendly acquaintances, or you may find that the relationship doesn't go anywhere. You may develop a relationship with a goddess that ends once your work together is done. Continue seeking patiently until you forge a connection.

SEEK
WISDOM

Bay leaves have long been associated with wisdom, and cauldrons with knowledge. You can go all out for this spell and use an iron cauldron for your brew, but it works just as well with a modern pot on the stove. Use this one when you seek deeper spiritual wisdom.

TIMING:

Lunar Phase: New Moon

Day: Any

YOU WILL NEED:

A handful of dried bay leaves

A mortar and pestle

1 to 2 cups of water in a pot on the stove

Milk and sugar to taste

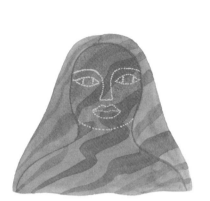

Crush the bay leaves into smaller tea leaves using the mortar and pestle. Bring the water to a boil and add the bay leaves. Boil for three minutes, stirring and inhaling the scent of the steam. Say:

Bay leaf, bay leaf, make me wise.
Bring me knowledge that I may rise.

Take the brew off the heat and pour it into a mug. Add plenty of milk and sugar to taste, since bay leaf tea is fairly bitter. Drink it, and when you are done, interpret the images in the tea leaves for signs from your working.

Look for signs and synchronicities over the next three days. You may meet someone or find out about an opportunity that could lead you further down your path.

DECLARE PERSONAL SOVEREIGNTY

Using spellwork for self-care is good for your physical and mental health, your relationships, and the wellbeing of your spirit, but most of all, it's about stepping into your own authority. When you do spellwork, you are the author of your own life. *Sovereignty*, your personal authority and self-governance, comes from the old French *soverain*, or "monarch." Empower yourself to rule your own life as the monarch of your domain.

TIMING:

Lunar Phase: Full Moon

Day: Any

YOU WILL NEED:

A crown, tiara, or headdress
that makes you feel regal

Dragon's blood incense

For this ritual, you will need a crown of some type. This can be a flower crown, a simple garland of ivy, a braid of ribbons, or an elaborate crown of crystals. You can make one yourself or purchase a piece that feels right. Aim for natural materials over synthetic. Dress in clothing that makes you feel powerful. Set your crown beside you, light the incense, and waft it around yourself as you say the following:

> I hereby declare myself
> A sovereign individual
> Bound to no one but myself
> And powerful beyond measure.

Place the crown on your head and feel your power flow into it. Surround yourself with protective light from the crown of your head, knowing that all of your magic comes from within you. You can wear this crown again when you need a reminder of your own sovereignty.

PLEDGE TO A
MORAL CODE

At times in your life, you will have to make decisions based on your personal moral code. This is a ritual for creating and sealing that code for yourself.

TIMING:

Any time

YOU WILL NEED:

A journal and a pen

Draw a vertical line down the center of a page in your journal. On the left-hand side, write "I will" and on the right-hand side write "I will not."

Under the first column, list things you will do with magic. The list of things you will do might include "empower myself," "help others," "create positive energy," or "heal."

The list of things you will not do might include "control others" and "hurt others." Think about circumstances in which you might override things on your "will not" list. Would you put a freezing spell on someone if you were in danger? That falls under the category of controlling others, but you would be doing it to protect yourself. Is it ethical for you? Be specific with your language.

Once you are satisfied with your list, write a moral code for yourself. Sign and date your pledge to this code and refer back to it when you need moral guidance.

Magical practitioners and pagans have different moral codes, depending on the traditions they practice. The moral code of the well-known Wiccan Rede is "An ye harm none, do what ye will." There are many ethical people who use magic for good, but witchcraft cannot be easily divided into "white magic" or "black magic." The ethics of magic are just like all other ethics: complex and sometimes murky.

INTEGRATE YOUR
SHADOW SIDE

Your shadow side is a part of you that represents
the aspects of yourself that you fear, dislike,
and would sometimes rather not acknowledge.
Your shadow might include jealousy, anger, egotism,
or greed. We are all human, and we all have
some darkness within us. That shadow of yours
has something to teach you. By acknowledging
your shadow and learning from it, you are
taking care of your whole self.

TIMING:

Lunar Phase: Waning Moon or New Moon

Day: Any

YOU WILL NEED:

A journal and a pen

A white candle

A black candle

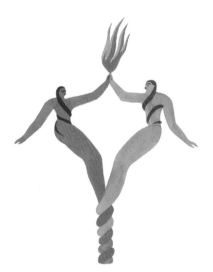

Find a comfortable seated position and close your eyes. Visualize yourself walking along a path in the woods. You come to a clearing, a circle of seven trees. In the middle of these trees is your shadow self. Notice what your shadow looks like. Walk up to your shadow and meet it face-to-face. Ask it what it has to teach you. Listen for the answer. When you are ready to leave, hug your shadow, thank yourself, and walk back down the path.

Open your eyes. Journal about what you have learned.

Put the white and black candles next to each other on your altar, so close that they touch each other, and light them, knowing that they are both a part of you, light and shadow. As they burn, the wax will melt together, symbolizing the integration of your whole self.

DEVELOP YOUR
INNER WARRIOR

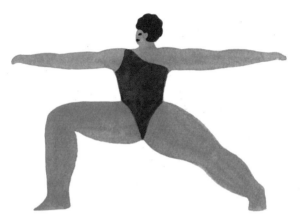

We all have Mars somewhere in our astrological chart, but womxn are discouraged from accessing the fiery, assertive, warrior strength of this planet. This is a ritual for developing your inner warrior so that you can draw on your courage to fight for what is important to you.

TIMING:

Lunar Phase: Waxing Moon or Full Moon

Day: Tuesday

YOU WILL NEED:

One red article of clothing or accessory
that can be worn while active

At least 4 red candles

Wearing your red piece of clothing or accessory, place the candles in a circle around you. Once you have prepared yourself and your space, light the candles. Say:

> I call on the energy of Mars,
> Courage, strength, will, and passion,
> To awaken within me the wise warrior,
> She who fights for what is right.

Envision yourself embodying assertiveness, passion, and strength.

Once this ritual is done, use your energy to do something physically active. Choose an activity that seems to activate your wise warrior energy. Developing your physical strength will help you to develop your inner strength.

Appendix

CORRESPONDENCES

—

Astrology and Timing

LUNAR PHASES

 New Moon: Good for setting intentions and the magic of new beginnings.

 Waxing Moon: Good for magic to do with growth and manifestation.

 Full Moon: Good for most magic, manifestation, and/or release.

 Waning Moon: Good for magic to do with release, banishing, or binding.

 Waning Crescent Moon: Especially good for banishing and binding magic.

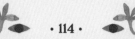

PLANETARY DAYS OF THE WEEK

Sunday: Sun. Success, joy, happiness, clarity, warmth.

Monday: Moon. Clairvoyance, emotions, spiritual connection.

Tuesday: Mars. Action, desire, passion, competition, vitality.

Wednesday: Mercury. Communication, messages, commerce, business.

Thursday: Jupiter. Good fortune, luck, abundance, wealth, spiritual connection.

Friday: Venus. Femininity, beauty, love, romance, self-care, abundance, wealth.

Saturday: Saturn. Protection, discipline, banishing, binding, consequences.

PLANETARY GLYPHS

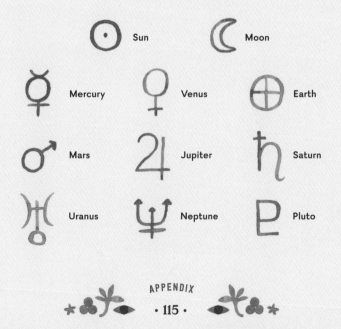

Sun

Moon

Mercury

Venus

Earth

Mars

Jupiter

Saturn

Uranus

Neptune

Pluto

Elements

Air: East. Intellect, communication, new beginnings, the dawn, travel, freedom, laughter.

Fire: South. Passion, desire, creativity, action, energy, will, strength, protection.

Water: West. Emotions, intuition, psychic powers, compassion, healing, cleansing, love.

Earth: North. Stability, fertility, prosperity, crops, nature, animals, strength, protection.

Colors

White: purity, innocence, spirituality. All-purpose color. Element: Water. Astrology: Moon.

Red: strength, passion, will, vitality, courage. Element: Fire. Astrology: Mars.

Orange: success, joy, creativity, vitality. Element: Fire. Astrology: Sun.

Yellow: communication, friendship, intellect, happiness. Element: Air. Astrology: Mercury, Sun.

Green: prosperity, abundance, growth, luck. Element: Earth. Astrology: Venus.

Blue: communication, good fortune, truth, harmony. Element: Water. Astrology: Jupiter, Moon.

Purple: wisdom, spiritual power, royalty, divinity. Element: Water. Astrology: Jupiter.

Pink: love, romance, healing, compassion, femininity. Element: Air. Astrology: Venus.

Black: protection, defense, banishing negativity, grounding. Element: Earth. Astrology: Saturn.

Plants, Herbs, and Essential Oils

Abre camino oil: banishing, clearing, protection, literally "opening the road"

Agrimony: banishing, protection, psychic shielding, healing, sleep

Argan oil: "liquid gold," health, beauty, life, vitality

Basil: success, love, money, peace, protection, purification

Bay leaves (bay laurel): psychic powers, healing, protection, banishing negativity, victory

Birch bark: new beginnings, birth, renewal, inner strength, psychic protection

Cayenne pepper: fidelity, love, warmth, protection, healing

Cedar: longevity, protection, preservation, growth, illumination

Cinnamon: love, happiness, money

Chocolate: love, romance, intimacy, power, virility

Cloves: purification, removal of negativity, protection, memory

✳ **Comfrey:** protection (especially for travel or from theft), healing, restoration

Dragon's blood: protection, manifestation, power

Echinacea: health, strength, energy, vitality

Fennel: protection, psychic protection, confidence, courage, communication, purification

Ginger: warmth, health, passion, fertility

Honeysuckle: prosperity, clairvoyance, protection

Hyssop: purification, cleansing, protection, healing

Jasmine: self-love, self-confidence, sensuality, prosperity

✳★ **Juniper:** protection, rejuvenation, energy, success, love

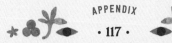

Lavender: peace, happiness, protection, love, friendship, harmony, cooperation

Lemon: cleansing, purification, health, love, good fortune

❋ **Mugwort:** protection, psychic vision, astral travel, wisdom

Orange: wealth, prosperity, joy, happiness, luck

Patchouli: attraction, protection, peace of mind, passion, love, prosperity, destiny

Peppermint: wisdom, money, luck, hospitality, healing

Raspberry: fertility, pregnancy, reproductive organs, protection, strength

Rose: love, romance, good luck, happiness, friendship

Rosemary: memory, protection, fidelity, love

Sage: longevity, prosperity, health, protection, cleansing, wisdom

Sandalwood: protection, purification, healing, stress relief

Sesame oil: energy, immortality, health, wisdom, luck

Tea tree: strength, harmony, protection, purification, clarity

Thyme: peace, tranquility, security, purification, clairvoyance

Vanilla: love, calm, mental awareness, personal empowerment, good luck

KEY

✳ Poisonous. Not safe to ingest.

❋ Safe in small doses, but toxic if overused.

★ Do not use if pregnant.

NOTE: Spell ingredients are chosen for their magical properties. The herbs, plants, and oils listed should be safe to use as directed in these spells. Check to make sure you're not allergic to an ingredient before ingesting it or using it on your skin. Always check with your doctor if you are pregnant or have a condition that may make some plants unsafe for you to use.

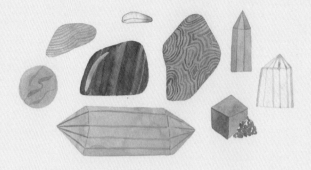

Crystals

Amazonite: courage, truth, integrity, authenticity

Amethyst: spiritual connection, calming, healing, mental focus

Aventurine: luck, prosperity, opportunity, motivation, perseverance

Blue lace agate: clarity, communication, encouragement, stability

Citrine: bliss, confidence, solar power, creativity, clarity

Hematite: grounding, banishing negativity, protection

Labradorite: healing, protection, clairvoyance, wisdom

Malachite: wealth, commerce, travel, protection

Rose quartz: love, compassion, healing, happiness, warmth

Selenite: psychic protection, clairvoyance, cleansing, healing

Tiger's eye: courage, energy, harmony, balance, protection, manifestation

DIVINATION METHODS

Pendulum

You can purchase a crystal pendulum at most of the magical supply stores listed in the Resources section (page 126), or you can use a necklace, cord, or chain with a crystal or bauble at the end. To use a pendulum, hold it by the top of the chain and ask a yes or no question. If it swings front to back, the answer is yes. If it swings side to side, the answer is no.

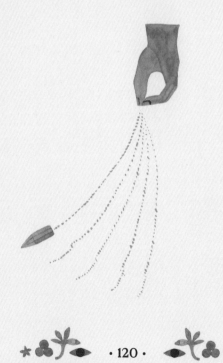

Runes

The runic alphabet is a sacred alphabet of symbols passed down from the Vikings. Runes were used as magical symbols for power, luck, and wealth. The ten runes listed here can be used in talismans, candle carvings, and other spells.

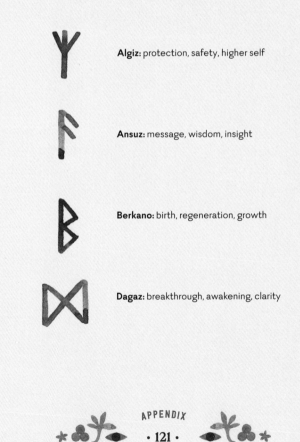

Algiz: protection, safety, higher self

Ansuz: message, wisdom, insight

Berkano: birth, regeneration, growth

Dagaz: breakthrough, awakening, clarity

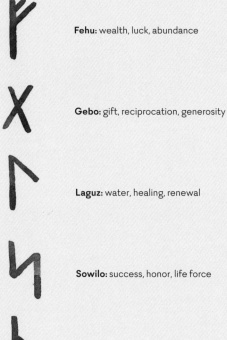

Fehu: wealth, luck, abundance

Gebo: gift, reciprocation, generosity

Laguz: water, healing, renewal

Sowilo: success, honor, life force

Thurisaz: will, regeneration, change

Wunjo: joy, harmony, comfort

 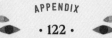

Scrying

Scrying is the art of telling the future through vision, most commonly by looking at a reflective surface like a crystal ball. Scrying can also be done by gazing into water, flames, smoke, or a mirror. To scry, relax your vision and gaze into the surface patiently. Interpret the visions that appear.

Tarot Cards

The tarot deck is a 78-card deck used to divine the future. All tarot decks have the same 22 Major Arcana cards, along with 56 other cards in the suits of swords, wands, cups, and pentacles. There are many tarot decks to choose from. Some of the most widely used include the Waite-Smith Tarot, the Thoth Tarot, and the Wildwood Tarot. Every deck comes with its own guide to the symbolism of the cards.

Some of the spells in this book include tarot cards. "Make New Friends" (page 69) calls for the Three of Cups and "Access Your Strength" (page 40) calls for the Strength card. You can find these in any tarot deck or print images from the internet for use in a spell.

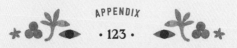

Tea Leaves

Reading tea leaves is another way to prophesy the future. Put a pinch of loose leaf tea in a mug and pour boiling water over it. Let it sit for three minutes or so. Drink the liquid, leaving just a little bit at the bottom, and interpret the shapes you see left by the leaves.

Animal Tracks

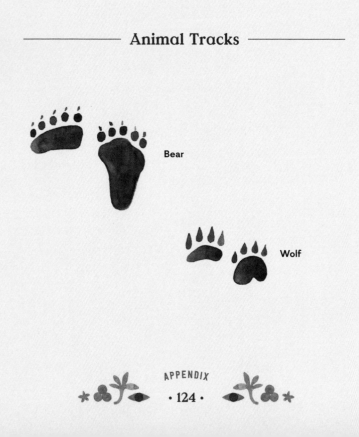

Bear

Wolf

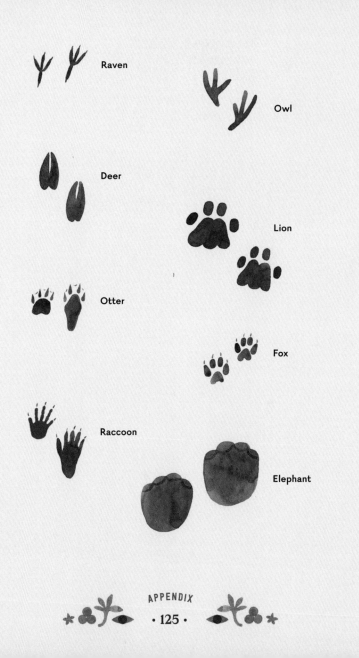

Raven

Owl

Deer

Lion

Otter

Fox

Raccoon

Elephant

RESORCES

These magical and metaphysical shops carry herbs, crystals, tarot cards, ritual tools, and more. Many also offer classes and gatherings. To find more shops in your area or online, search witchvox.com.

CHICAGO

Alchemy Arts
1203 W. Bryn Mawr Ave.
Chicago, IL 60660
(773) 769-4970
alchemy-arts.com

LOS ANGELES

The Green Man
5712 Lankershim Blvd.
North Hollywood, CA 91601
(818) 985-2010
thegreenmanstore.com

NEW YORK

Enchantments
424 East 9th St.
New York, NY 10009
(212) 228-4394
enchantmentsincnyc.com

OAKLAND, CA

Ancient Ways
4075 Telegraph Ave.
Oakland, CA 94609
(510) 653-3244
ancientways.com

ONLINE ONLY

13 Moons Magical Supplies
13moons.com

Grove and Grotto
groveandgrotto.com

The Magickal Cat
themagickalcat.com

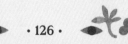

BIBLIOGRAPHY

Beck, Martha. "The 4-Step Plan to Get Your Life on Track."
Oprah.com. http://www.oprah.com/money/find-your-career-path/
all. Accessed August 3, 2018.

Bromius, Ivy. "The Agile Manifesto." Circle Thrice.
https://circlethrice.com. Accessed June 16, 2018.

Castellano, Deborah. *Glamour Magic: The Witchcraft Revolution to
Get What You Want.* Woodbury, MN: Llewellyn Worldwide, 2017.

Cunningham, Scott. *The Complete Book of Incense, Oils, and Brews.*
Woodbury, MN: Llewellyn, 1989.

Miller, Jason. *Protection and Reversal Magick.* New Jersey: New
Page Books, 2006.

———. *Financial Sorcery: Magical Strategies to Create Real and
Lasting Wealth.* New Jersey: New Page Books, 2012.

National Heart, Lung, and Blood Institute. "Sleep Deprivation and
Deficiency." https://www.nhlbi.nih.gov/health-topics/sleep-
deprivation-and-deficiency. Accessed August 3, 2018.

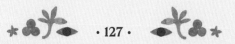

Ryan, Lisa. "You'll Never Guess Who Has the Most Orgasms."
The Cut (February 23, 2017). https://www.thecut.com/2017/02/
straight-men-orgasm-more-often-than-women-study.html.
Accessed August 3, 2018.

Taleb, Nicholas Nassim. *Antifragile: Things That Gain from Disorder.*
New York: Random House, 2012.

Thorpe, JR. "Why Self-Care Is an Important Feminist Act."
Bustle (December 16, 2014). https://www.bustle.com/
articles/200074-why-self-care-is-an-important-feminist-act.
Accessed August 3, 2018.

White, Gordon. Rune Soup. https://runesoup.com. Accessed
August 3, 2018.

Wood, Jamie. *The Teen Spell Book: Magick for Young Witches.*
New York: Celestial Arts, 2001.

———. *The Wicca Herbal: Recipes, Magick, and Abundance.*
New York: Celestial Arts, 2003.

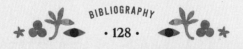